A Couple's SURVIVAL Guide to Menopause

Navigate perimenopause symptoms together
Know what he wants and she needs

First Published in Australia in 2024 by Sobrietea Pty Ltd

Copyright © 2024 by Samantha Siân Brown

The moral right of the author has been asserted.

Illustrations and Cover copyright Kylie Dunn

All rights reserved.

No part of this publication may be reproduced, stored in a retrieval system, or transmitted in any form or by any means, without the prior permission in writing of the publisher, nor be otherwise circulated in any form of binding or cover other than that in which it is published and without a similar condition including this condition being imposed on the subsequent purchaser. This includes the exclusion of using or reproducing this book in any manner for the purpose of training artificial intelligence technologies or systems.

ISBN: 978-1-7635667-0-5

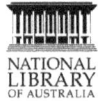 A catalogue record for this book is available from the National Library of Australia

Printed and bound in Australia, United States or United Kingdom by IngramSpark, Lightning Source Inc.

Dedication

For all the women who have lost their former body shape, resilience, mental acuity, sleep, libido, keen memory, sense of direction, and more—I see you.

For all the caring and confounded male partners who want to understand what's going on and how to help—I see you too.

Disclaimer

The information provided in this book is intended for general informational and educational purposes only. It does not constitute professional medical, psychological, or any other form of advice. The author and publisher are not qualified to provide such professional services and therefore do not offer or imply any guarantees or assurances. Readers should consult with a qualified health professional for advice tailored to their individual circumstances. Reliance on any information contained in this book is solely at your own risk. The author and publisher accept no responsibility for any errors, omissions, or consequences arising from the use of this information.

CONTENTS

Preface	1
Key Definitions	4
1. Sex	7
2. Temperature	11
3. Moods	14
4. Memory	18
5. Joints	22
6. Body Shape	26
7. Diet & Exercise	30
8. Periods	34
9. Bone Density	38
10. HRT	42
Detailed Definitions	46
Epilogue	50
Acknowledgements	52
About the Author	53

Preface

I had just turned 50, and in the pre-dawn hours, I was consumed by yet another hot flash. Feeling frustrated and bone-deep tired after enduring another night of broken sleep, my thoughtful partner picked up his Formula One racing car magazine and began to fan me. The effect was wonderfully cooling, but it also sent me into a fit of sleep-deprived hysteria. It was in this moment—his act of caring and my sudden revelation that menopause is a maelstrom and a mystery to many—that the idea for this book was born.

In that truly intimate moment, I realised that couples, not just women, needed to understand what is going on during perimenopause, and how supportive partners, bewildered by the symptoms, could help if only they knew how.

With the car magazine returned to the bedside table and a cup of tea in hand, I grabbed a notepad and listed my perimenopause symptoms: hot flashes, sleep loss, brain fog, increased irritability, tearfulness, erratic periods, low libido, rapid weight gain, persistent joint pain, loss of motivation, and… quite a lot of grumpiness. Although I had read or listened to numerous detailed (and somewhat depressing) books on menopause, I decided to research perimenopause symptoms beyond those I was already familiar with. I found that increased anxiety, heavy bleeding, reduced capacity to cope, forgetfulness, hair loss, malaise, and—what I now call the 'silent symptom'—osteoporosis were common among women typically over 40, with any or all these symptoms lasting an average of 4-8 years. Cripes!

But where was the introductory guide to help us understand this phase we call 'menopause'? I considered that both women and men should have something easily digestible on the 'what and why' of perimenopause and menopause. Many women like me are leading very busy lives, often in management positions, with teenage kids, aging parents, and a 'perimenopause brain', thus minimising the appetite for reading a lengthy 'War and Peace on menopause'. Men, generally, are unlikely to read anything on menopause, so something short, informative, and illustrated might just be the 'snack-size' he'd be willing to read. I'm hoping it's even succinct enough for him to read cover to cover in one sitting!

So, this book was created with five principles in mind:

- For women and men
- Short
- Informative
- Shareable
- Funny

This book was never intended to be a comprehensive deep dive into the complexities of perimenopause, menopause, and post-menopause, nor does it include detailed endocrinology or exhaustive psychology. Instead, it has been simply designed to help you learn the basic facts, pick up some pointers about each other, and share a laugh together.

My intention was to help couples cope better together and maintain their relationship through and beyond her 'change of life.'

I will, however, admit that I've done so with some tongue-in-cheek humour (he wants, she needs) and a bit of gender stereotyping, but I stand by my goal: this guidebook is here to help you both, and as a couple, survive the perimenopause years together.

With all that said, along with my caring, thoughtful, supportive, and ever-amorous partner, we were determined to make it to the other side of my transition with understanding, humour, ongoing intimacy, and most importantly, an intact relationship.

And we want that for you too.

All the best,

Samantha

The author of this book is she/her and her partner is he/him. The context of this book is of a heterosexual nature. No offence was intended in the writing and/or depictions created in this guide despite some stereotyping that is portrayed.

Note also, for the purposes of this book the term 'woman' or 'women' refers to a person(s) who has/had dominant hormones of estrogen and progesterone and has, or had, a uterus and ovaries, and is (typically) over the age of 40 experiences some, or all, of the physical and mental changes commonly referred to as perimenopause or menopause symptoms.

Key Definitions

Perimenopause

A natural phase in woman's life, usually commencing in her early to mid-40's. May last several months or up to a decade, but typically 4-8 years. The symptoms outlined in this book are common perimenopausal symptoms.

Menopause

A specific point in time, after which a woman has gone 12 months consecutively without having a period. On average this happens at age 51.

Note: Commonly what people call 'menopause' is in fact the phase and symptoms of perimenopause.

Post Menopause

The phase of life after the point of menopause, until death.

Hot flash/Hot flush

Brief experiences of increased heat, typically in the upper torso, neck and face, that last from thirty seconds up to several minutes.

HRT

Hormone Replacement Therapy. *See Detailed Definitions on page 46 for more information.*

THE MENOPAUSE TIMELINE

Figure 1. The timeline of perimenopause to post menopause, punctuated by menopause.

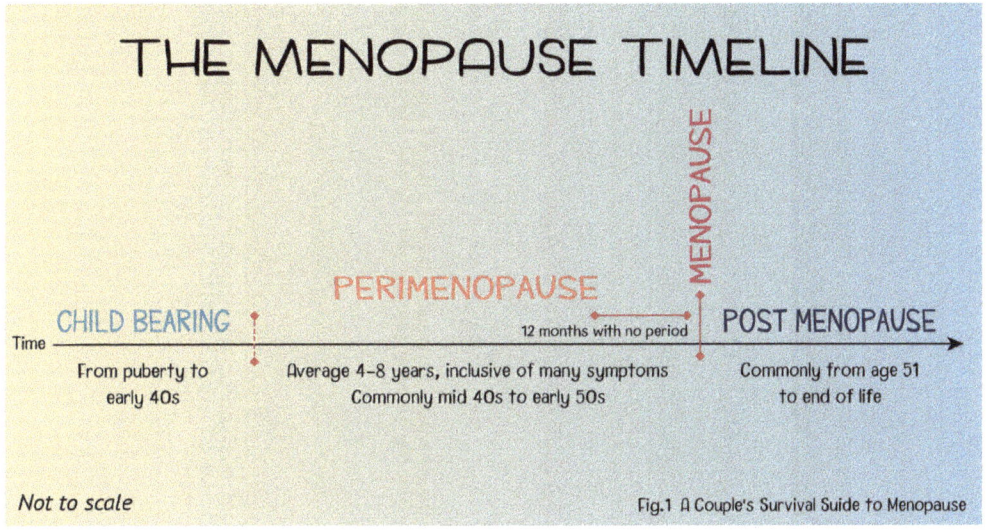

1. Sex

Once upon a time you were both up for it, every night, twice even thrice, but now, not so much…

What's going on?

During perimenopause and menopause, women often face significant physiological and emotional changes that can impact their inclination towards intimacy with their partner.

Physiologically, hormonal fluctuations lead to decreased estrogen levels, resulting in symptoms like vaginal dryness and discomfort during intercourse, making sexual activity less appealing. These hormonal changes can also cause tender breasts, adding physical discomfort to the mix, and lead to erratic periods, introducing an element of unpredictability that can further disrupt sexual intimacy. Other symptoms, such as hot flashes, sleep disturbances, fatigue, and weight gain, further decrease libido by affecting body image and overall physical well-being.

Emotionally, the transition into menopause can be challenging. Mood swings, anxiety, and depression due to hormonal changes can affect a woman's desire for intimacy. The psychological impact of aging and societal perceptions of menopause as the end of fertility can also negatively influence a woman's self-image and sexual desire.

These physiological and emotional shifts can create a tumultuous period for a woman, making the prospect of intimacy less appealing.

What he wants

- All nighters, like when they first met.
- The freedom to have sex without the complication of erratic periods.
- Spontaneity without the requirement for lube.
- No limits on breast fondling due to tenderness.
- For her not to stress about her weight gain and loss of feeling young and sexy.

What she needs

- No pressure or expectations that intimacy will be as frequent, raunchy or spontaneous as before.
- No groping when she has tender breasts.
- To wear fluffy PJs to bed and still be held with affection (until she has a hot flash).
- Not to be prodded in the night by his hard-on after she has just got back to sleep after yet another night sweat.
- Understanding and patience whilst she is navigating a raft of unwelcome and uncertain physical and mental changes.

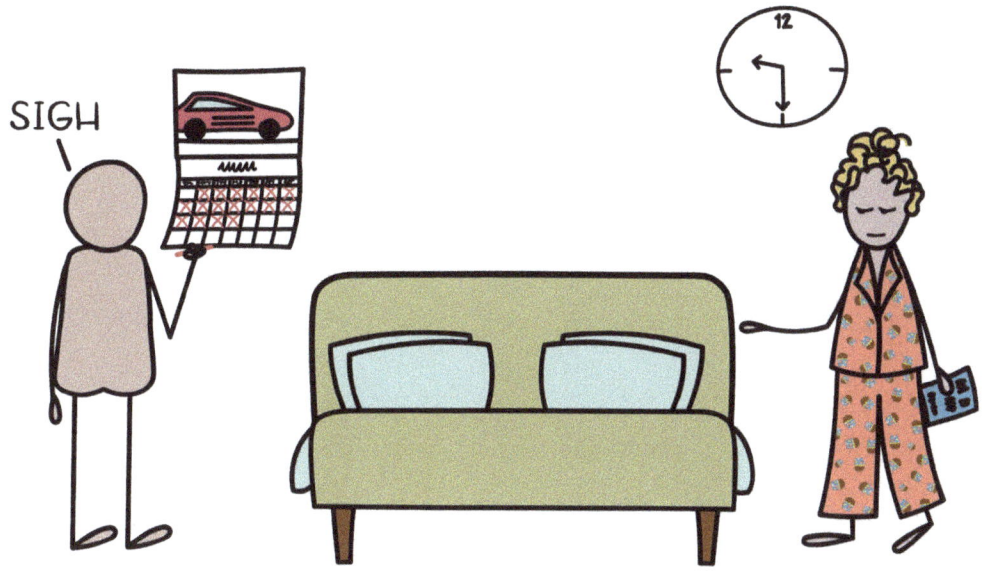

2. Temperature

Sometimes she runs hotter than a V8 at the Bathurst 1000 Supercar Championships!

What's going on?

During menopause, a woman's body experiences a notable decline in estrogen, leading to disruptions in internal temperature regulation. This hormonal imbalance affects the hypothalamus, the body's thermostat, causing it to malfunction.

Women may experience hot flashes which are sudden intense heat surges across the upper body, lasting from thirty seconds to several minutes, due to dilated blood vessels near the skin's surface, causing redness and often sweating as a cooling mechanism.

Night sweats, the nocturnal counterpart, significantly disrupt sleep, leading to sleep deprivation that can exacerbate mood swings, memory issues, weight gain, and decreased libido.

Note also that these sweats can occur during the day and may persist even after menopause, highlighting the enduring impact of hormonal changes on a woman's body and well-being.

What he wants

- Closeness and cuddle times that aren't governed by interruptive hot flashes.
- Fair half (or more) of the mattress.
- To not have to change the sheets during the night.
- Her nakedness to lead to intimacy (not just because she is too hot for night-clothes).

What she needs

- Space in the bed to move to a cool zone.
- No objections to the doona/duvet going on and off unpredictably.
- To be brought glasses of very cold water.
- To be brought a cool damp face washer.
- To be fanned.
- Acceptance that she's not in control of the heat fluctuations.
- Patience and respect if she suddenly pulls away from contact.
- Willingness to do extra washing.
- No objections to car windows being opened unexpectedly.
- Freedom to suddenly strip off clothes without the expectation of intimacy.

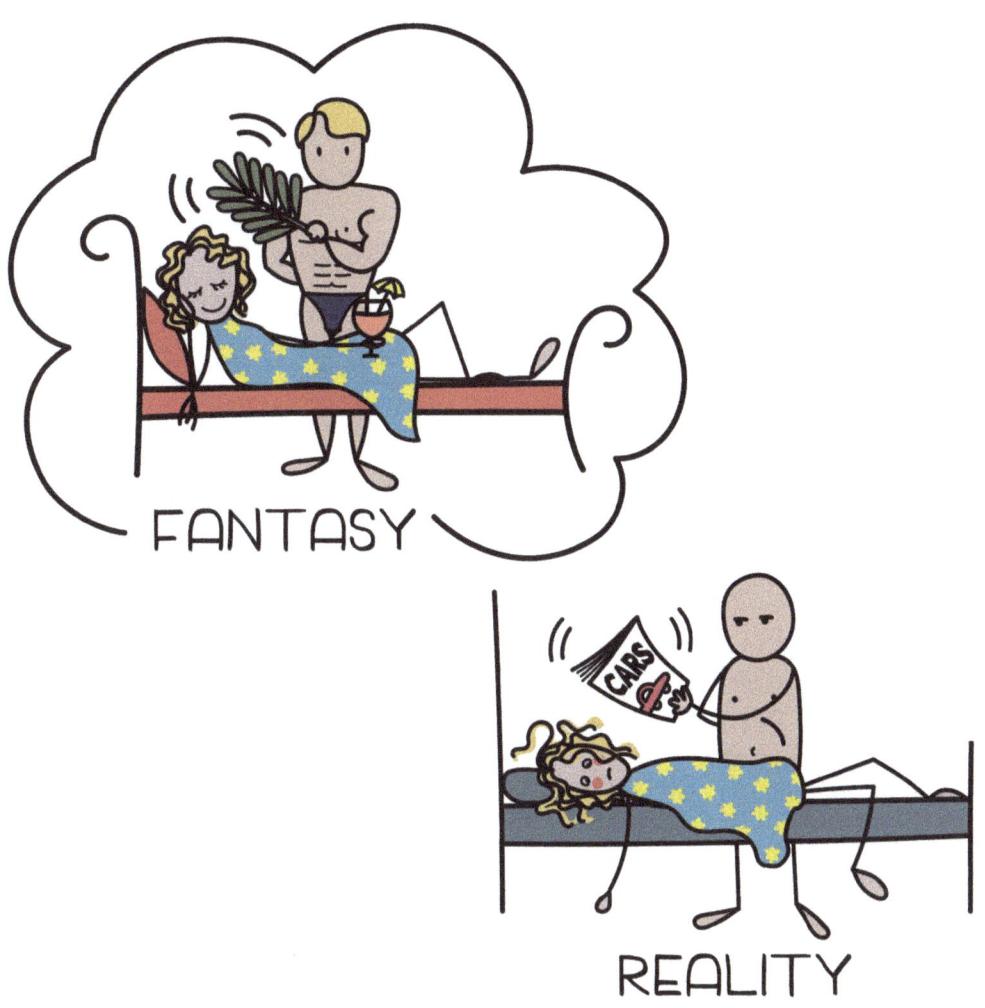

3. Moods

Like the weather in Tasmania, Australia come back in half an hour to find something different!

What's going on?

During menopause, the decline in estrogen significantly affects a woman's mood, due to its role beyond reproductive health—it influences mood-regulating neurotransmitters like serotonin and noradrenalin (norepinephrine). As estrogen decreases, the balance of these chemicals shifts, causing mood swings, irritability, and heightened stress sensitivity. Serotonin, crucial for well-being and happiness, and noradrenalin, which governs focus and stress response, are both impacted, making emotional regulation more challenging.

Progesterone and testosterone also diminish during this phase. Progesterone's reduction is notable since it naturally calms the brain and alleviates anxiety, whereas testosterone's drop can affect vitality, lowering energy and motivation. The adrenal glands attempt to offset these hormonal losses by increasing cortisol production, further amplifying stress responses.

Moreover, estrogen's influence on dopamine, the neurotransmitter associated with pleasure, means its decrease can dull enjoyment and satisfaction, exacerbating mood issues. Coupled with chronic sleep disturbances, common during menopause, these hormonal and neurotransmitter changes form a complex network that can significantly disrupt a woman's mood and emotional state.

What he wants:

- Calmness
- Rationality
- Predictability

What she needs:

- More rest and guilt free opportunities to sit down with a book or take a bath or shower.
- Understanding and patience when she isn't being as mindful or controlled as you may be accustomed to.
- Good communication including acts of forgiveness.
- Quality sleep. Don't prod her awake for sex if she has been woken up multiple times with hot flashes.
- Support when she is overwhelmed, unmotivated, tired, grumpy and disenchanted.

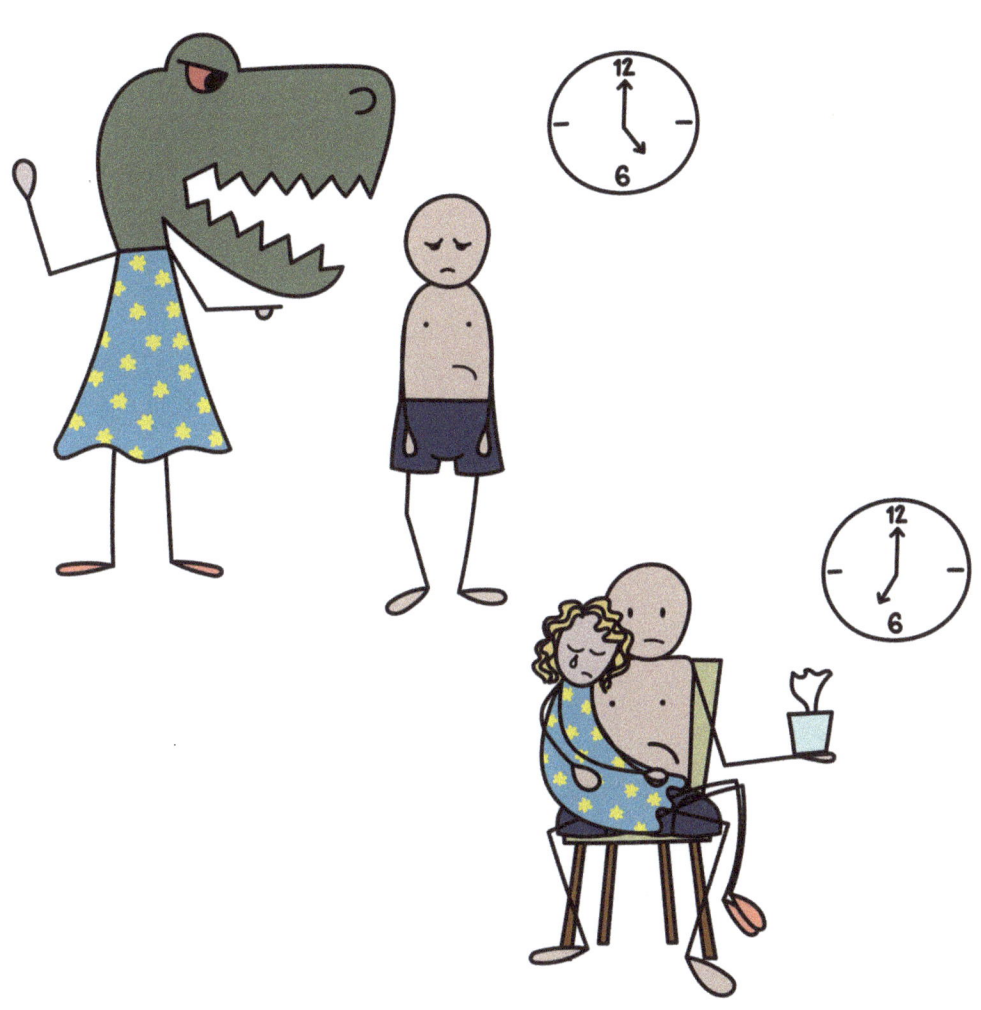

4. Memory

It's probably not early onset dementia, but at times menopause related memory loss appears a lot like it.

What's going on?

During perimenopause, women undergo significant hormonal shifts, especially in estrogen and progesterone levels. These changes directly influence cognitive functions, notably memory. Estrogen is particularly crucial for brain health, aiding in memory formation and retrieval processes. Moreover, perimenopause often brings disrupted sleep patterns—insomnia, sleep disturbances, and night sweats—further impacting memory. These sleep issues impede the brain's ability to consolidate memories effectively.

Additionally, many women report experiencing 'brain fog' during this time, a state characterised by confusion, forgetfulness, and a lack of focus and clarity. This phenomenon can be attributed to the hormonal imbalances that affect cognitive functions, making it challenging to process information as efficiently as usual.

Together, hormonal fluctuations and poor sleep quality form a challenging environment for cognitive health during menopause, leading to memory difficulties and brain fog. These symptoms are distinct from normal age-related cognitive changes, underscoring the unique impact of menopause on women's cognitive well-being.

What he wants

- Conversations without repetition.
- Not to be forgotten, including his name.
- For things/events/appointments not to be forgotten.
- For her not to be frustrated by her own memory loss and feeling down on herself about it.

What she needs

- Patience and understand that memory lapses are part of hormonal changes.
- Supportive communication with attentive listening without judgment.
- Practical assistance with gentle reminders about tasks or appointments without judgment.
- Empathy and emotional reassurance that memory lapses don't define her.
- Working together to reduce stress.
- Guilt free time to relax and unwind.
- No judgement on the wine/gin the night before.

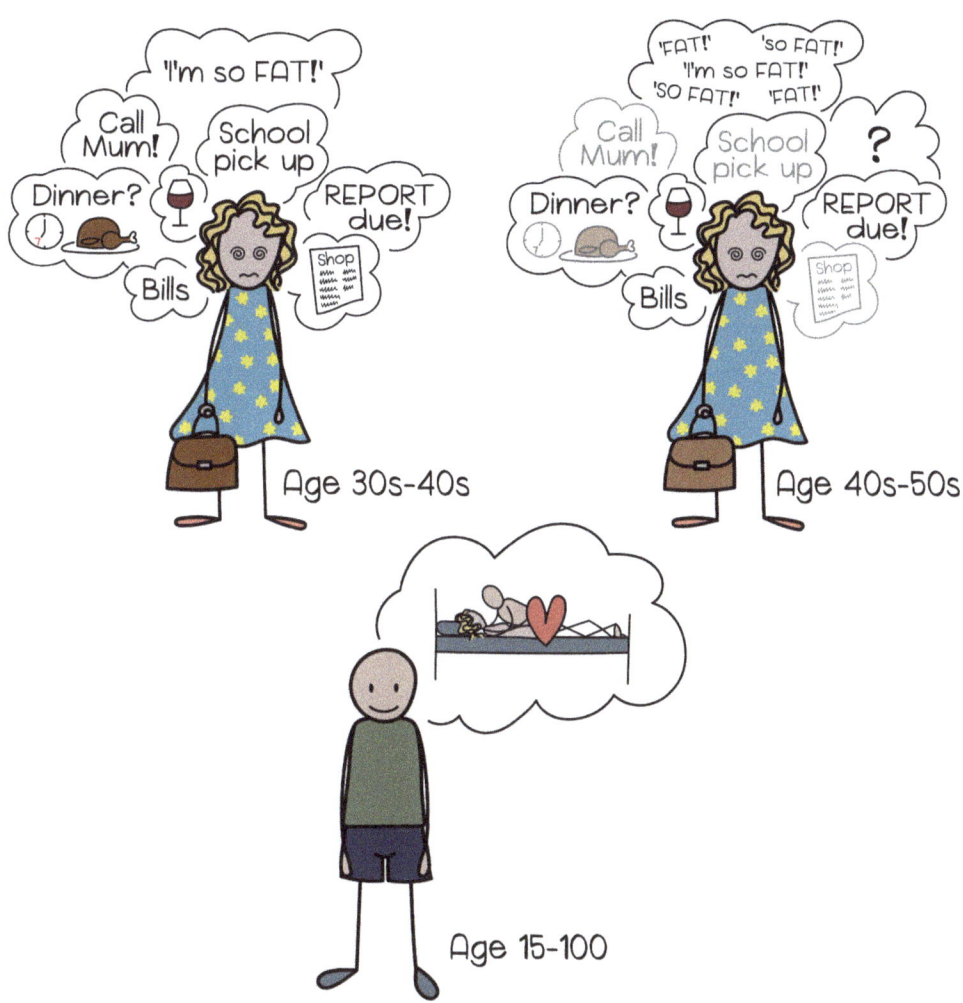

5. Joints

She is barely 50 years old yet can feel closer to 100! Commonly, at least one major joint is painful for months yet without any evidence of injury.

What's going on?

During perimenopause and menopause, women often experience increased joint pain due to the significant decline in estrogen levels. Estrogen is vital for joint health, as it regulates inflammation, aids in collagen production, and maintains the elasticity of ligaments and tendons. With lower estrogen, joints become less flexible, inflammation rises, and the risk of conditions like bursitis increases.

These hormonal changes, alongside the menopausal redistribution of body fat, place additional strain on joints. The knees, supporting much of the body's weight, face heightened strain, while hips, crucial for mobility, experience discomfort from altered joint fluidity. Wrists and shoulders, integral to many daily activities, also suffer from reduced flexibility and increased inflammation.

Estrogen functions like joint oil, and its decline causes joints to become more susceptible to discomfort and damage, akin to a car engine running without sufficient oil.

What he wants

- Not to see her in pain and unable to enjoy a range of activities.
- Keeping previous lifestyle and exercise routines intact.
- No Zimmer frames.

What she needs

- An explanation why her joints feel like they're falling apart, or someone is stabbing them.
- Understanding, compassion and support from friends, family and workplace; it is hard to cope with ongoing joint pain, while juggling everything else.
- Quality pain relief without side effects.
- Guilt free rest.
- To be brought hot packs, ice packs, pain relief and large glasses of wine/gin whilst remaining on the couch with her feet up.

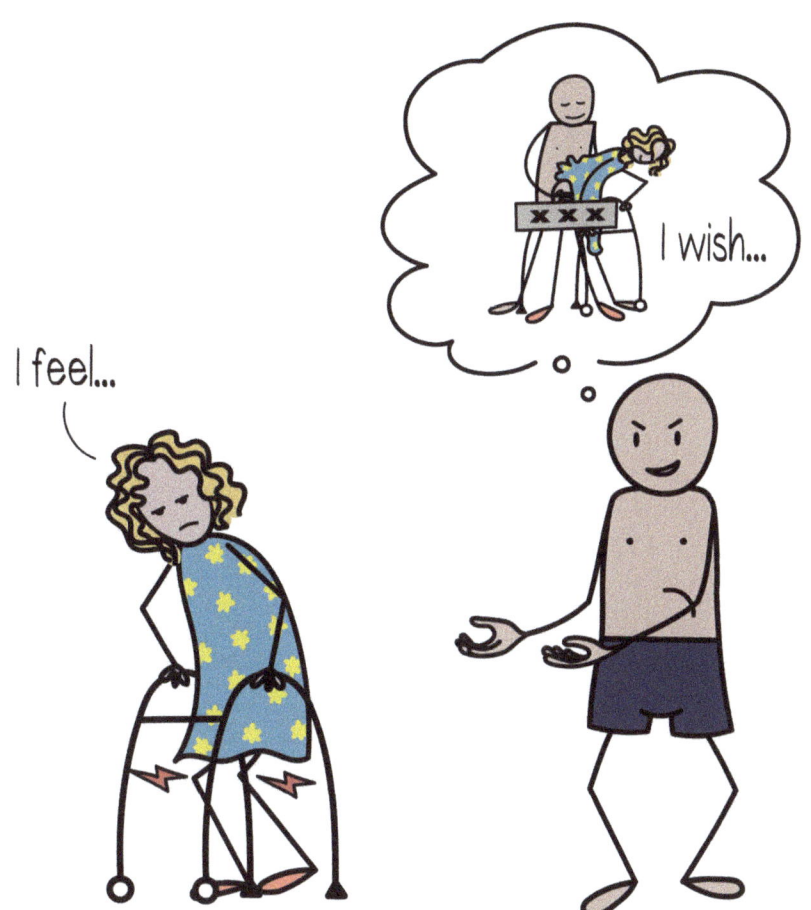

6. Body Shape

Pregnant? No! Enlarged breasts? Yes!

What's going on?

Estrogen plays a crucial role in regulating body fat distribution and metabolism. When estrogen levels decline for women in perimenopause and menopause, several physiological changes occur that can lead to weight gain:

Metabolic Rate: Estrogen helps regulate metabolic rate, the rate at which the body burns calories for energy. As estrogen levels decrease, metabolic rate may also decline, leading to fewer calories burned at rest.

Fat Storage: Estrogen influences where fat is stored in the body. Higher estrogen levels tend to favour fat deposition in the hips and thighs (pre-perimenopause years), while lower levels result in more fat being stored in the abdomen and bust.

Appetite Regulation: Estrogen plays a role in appetite regulation by affecting the levels of neurotransmitters involved in hunger and satiety signals. When estrogen levels drop, appetite may increase, leading to overeating and weight gain.

Insulin Sensitivity: Estrogen helps maintain insulin sensitivity, which is the body's ability to respond to insulin and regulate blood sugar levels. Lower estrogen levels can lead to insulin resistance, promoting fat storage, particularly in the abdominal region.

Water Retention: Hormonal changes can also influence fluid retention in the body. This may cause temporary bloating and the swelling of breast tissue.

Changes in breast tissue composition: A decrease in glandular tissue and an increase in fatty tissue can affect breast size and shape, usually by several increases in bra size.

What he wants

- A woman that doesn't bemoan her new fatter shape every moment of the day and night.
- A woman that still enjoys being naked around him.

What she needs

- Understanding that the increases in belly fat and breast size is due to the body's natural perimenopause process.
- Understanding that she has a changed metabolism due to age and hormonal changes.
- Not to be told to exercise more and harder.
- Not to be told drink less wine/gin (even if that could be beneficial).
- To be genuinely admired with all her new curves.
- Permission to buy bigger bras and clothes that she feels comfortable in (and/or sexy in).
- To be compassionately listened to when she is upset about other people's judgment.

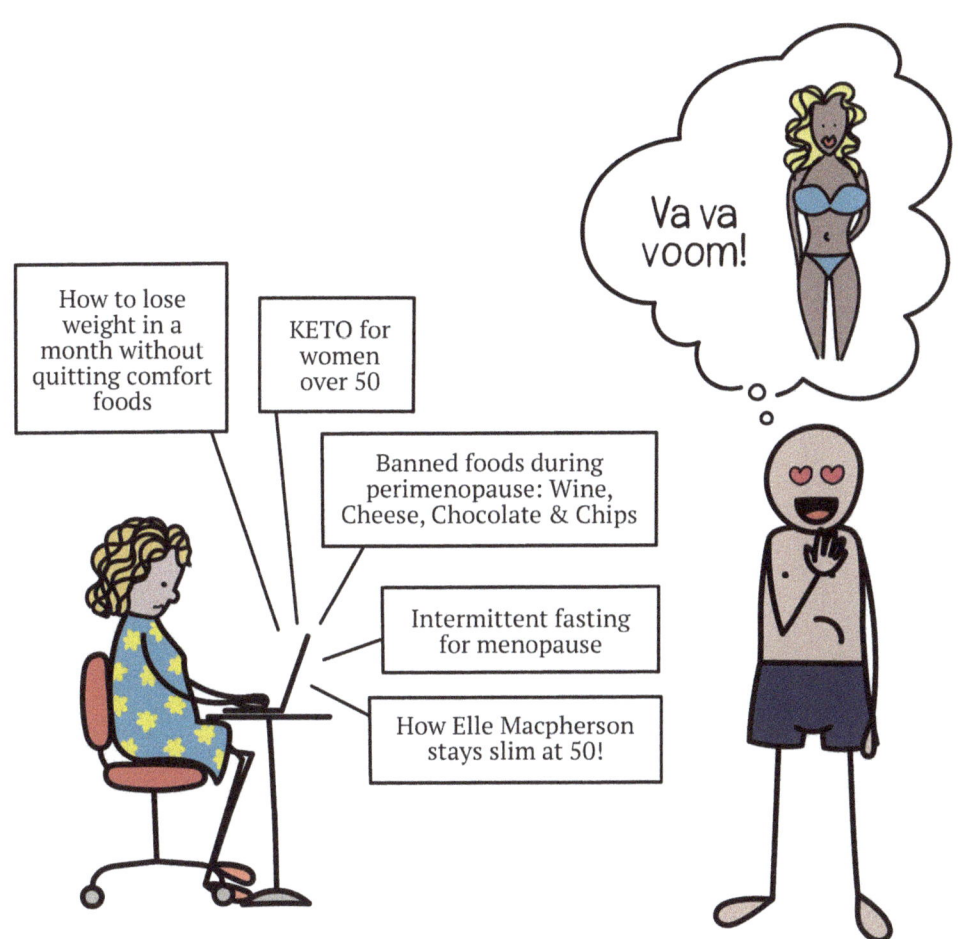

7. Diet & Exercise

From a racetrack mare to a plump paddock pony, all attempts at (previously successful) diets and exercise no longer bring the results.

What's going on?

Women in perimenopause and menopause experience significant hormonal changes that can slow down metabolism, decrease muscle mass, and alter fat distribution, presenting unique dietary and exercise challenges.

Traditional low-fat diets might not be the best choice during this stage since they often lack the essential healthy fats needed for maintaining hormonal balance. Diets that heavily restrict certain macronutrients can upset hormonal equilibrium and increase stress. Additionally, Intermittent Fasting can introduce extra stress and elevated cortisol levels, which might negatively impact sleep quality and hormonal balance, potentially undermining weight loss efforts.

Exercise preferences may also need adjustment. Cardio-centric exercises, for instance, can elevate cortisol levels, which might contribute to increased abdominal fat without effectively combating muscle loss.

Additionally, joint pain, a common issue discussed previously, can limit the ability to engage in certain physical activities.

To navigate these challenges, adopting low-impact exercises such as yoga, Pilates, Qi Gong, walking, and water-based activities, along with strength training, would be beneficial. Reducing the intake of processed foods, caffeine, and alcohol can also help.

Embracing diets like the Mediterranean or DASH (Dietary Approaches to Stop Hypertension), which focus on nutritional density through fruits, vegetables, whole grains, lean proteins, and healthy fats, supports hormonal health. Plant-rich and low-glycaemic index foods, emphasising fibre and blood sugar stability, can aid in managing satiety and mood fluctuations.

What he wants

- To share in the same eating habits and training routines they previously enjoyed together.
- Maintain a sense of unity with shared goals in fitness and health.

What she needs

- No pressure to return to and persist with past routines that are no longer effective.
- Acceptance and love as she tries and adopts new health routines.
- A shared journey of health and open to new paths together.
- Understanding and support through her body's changes.
- No guilt for attending (sometimes sporadically) different yoga or other exercise classes as trials.

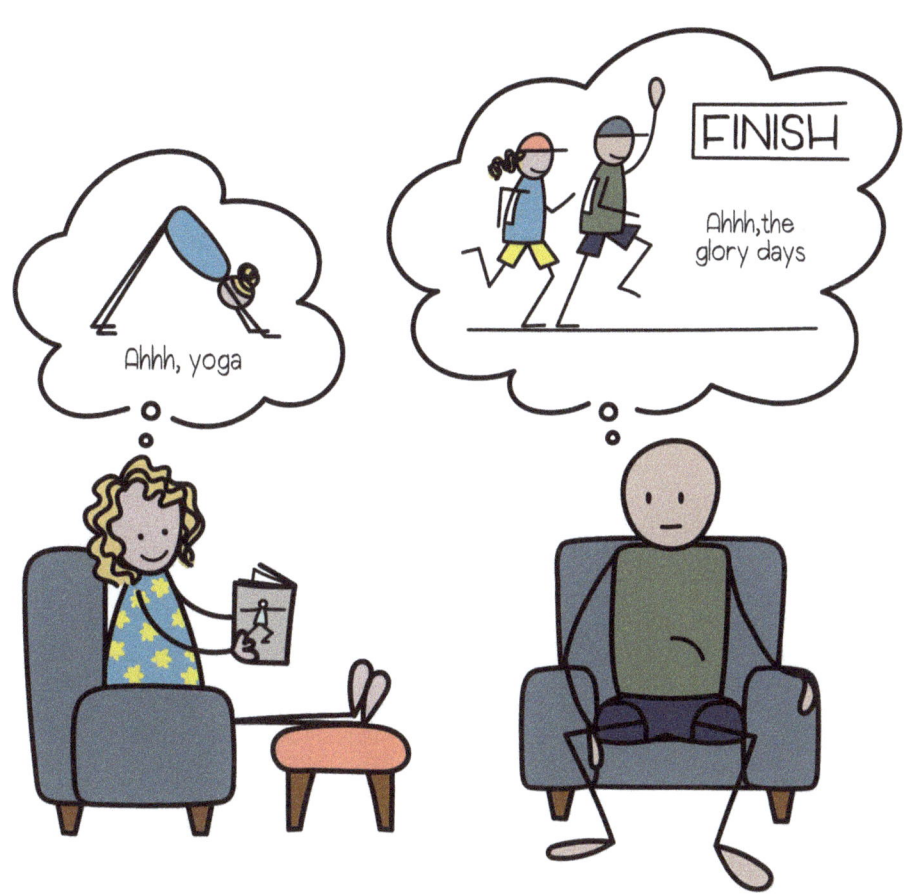

8. Periods

Once, a monthly routine with almost no fuss, her period has now become a force majeure.

What's going on?

During the transition from perimenopause to menopause, significant fluctuations in the body's production of estrogen and progesterone disrupt the regularity of menstrual cycles, leading to periods becoming irregular.

While a woman is still having periods, she remains in the perimenopausal phase. Hormonal fluctuations cause inconsistencies in the buildup and shedding of the endometrial lining, resulting in variability in menstrual blood volume, from very heavy bleeding to lighter periods or spotting.

Women in this phase often experience a range of emotions, such as fear when confronted with 'golf ball-sized blood clots,' frustration with irregular spotting, and annoyance with periods that can last for several weeks. They may also feel uncertain if they go several months without menstruation, only to have their hopes of reaching the '12-month amenorrhea' phase dashed by an unexpected spotting or heavy flow. Tiredness is exacerbated by these unpredictable and variable menstruation experiences.

As the phase of perimenopause progresses, the ovaries gradually reduce their production of estrogen and progesterone, decreasing fertility and eventually the cessation of all menstrual bleeding.

The hallmark point of reaching 'menopause' is defined as the moment a woman has completed a full 12 consecutive months without a period. During that 12 months she may or may not know if a period is pending, so the declaration of 'menopause' can only be made after the fact (12 months of no menstruation). Following this point, she enters 'post menopause'.

(See Key Definitions and Fig. 1 The Menopause Timeline)

What he wants

- Less erratic menstruation for easier planning of activities and life together.
- Less uncertainty on when (and if) she is menstruating, and for how many days and how heavy or light.
- A quick transition from periods to no periods, with no fuss.

What she needs

- Ways to manage and predict irregular menstrual cycles more effectively.
- Relief from symptoms like heavy bleeding or spotting.
- Options for hormonal or natural remedies to stabilise menstrual changes.
- Support and understanding from her partner, family and workplace as she navigates this variability and unpredictability.
- A period tracker app to keep records, including that all important 12 months without a period.

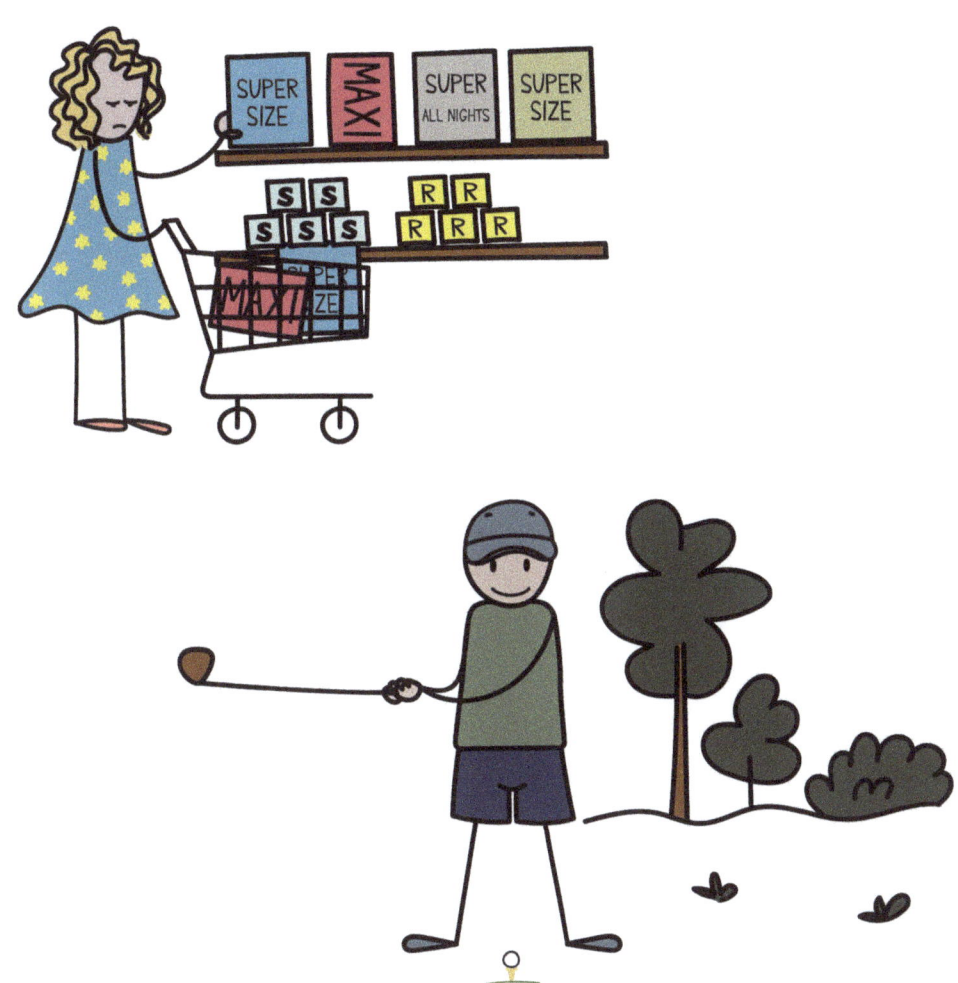

9. Bone Density

No, not his bone density, hers! The silent assassin – reduced bone density.

What's going on?

During perimenopause, the decrease in estrogen levels can lead to a reduction in bone density, increasing the risk of osteoporosis and fractures.

Estrogen plays a crucial role in maintaining bone density by helping to balance the bone remodelling process, where old bone is replaced with new bone tissue.

Additionally, estrogen is essential for efficient calcium absorption in the intestines, a process critical for bone health. As estrogen levels drop, not only does the rate of bone breakdown exceed the rate of bone formation, but calcium absorption can also diminish, leading to thinner, weaker bones.

To manage this risk, individuals are advised to engage in regular weight-bearing and muscle-strengthening exercises, maintain a diet rich in calcium and vitamin D, and avoid smoking and excessive alcohol consumption. In some cases, healthcare providers may recommend medications to protect bone health or hormone replacement therapy (HRT) to help mitigate the loss of bone density.

What he wants
- No frailty.
- More dates to drink milk shakes, eat ice cream and chocolate together.

What she needs
- Understanding this is a real risk to her health even though it's invisible.
- Calcium without the cholesterol and calories.
- A sustainable strength-based work out she enjoys.

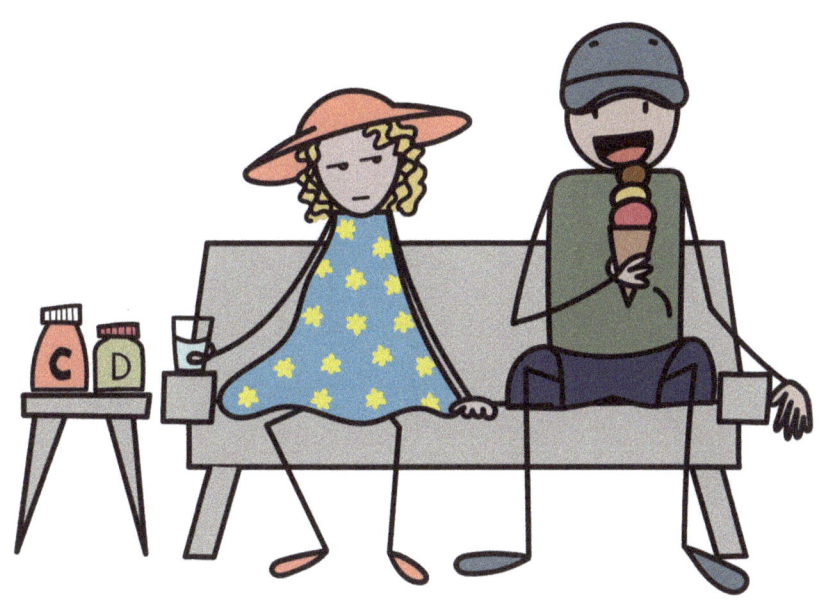

10. HRT

No, sorry, not the Holden Racing Team but Hormone Replacement Therapy as an option for woman to reduce the myriad of perimenopausal symptoms.

What, Why, Who, When

Hormone Replacement Therapy (HRT) is a treatment used to alleviate symptoms of perimenopause, a transitional phase before menopause.

During perimenopause, women experience fluctuations in hormone levels, particularly estrogen and progesterone, leading to symptoms like hot flashes, night sweats, joint pain, erratic periods, low libido, memory fog, weight gain, mood swings, and sleep disturbances.

HRT aims to balance these hormone levels by providing estrogen or a combination of estrogen and progesterone. This therapy can be administered through various forms, including pills, patches, gels, and creams.

The decision to start HRT is made on an individual basis, considering the woman's health history, symptom severity, and personal preferences. It's essential to consult with a healthcare provider to discuss the benefits and risks of HRT, as it may not be suitable for everyone.

Regular follow-ups and adjustments to the treatment plan are crucial to ensure the best outcome and minimise potential risks.

HRT can be initiated when perimenopause symptoms first appear and may continue into post-menopause, with the duration varying based on individual needs and medical advice.

What he wants

- No hocus-pocus.
- A quick return to the 'normal' woman he was in a relationship with before her hormones started changing.
- To understand if HRT increases or decreases the chances of pregnancy.
- To understand if HRT increases or decreases her libido.

What she needs

- Patience and a good listener as she navigates the information for and against HRT.
- Compassion if she chooses to trial HRT and is challenged by her symptoms and side effects whilst she gets the dosage right.
- Respect if she chooses not to trial HRT.
- Patience if she chooses to go off HRT and symptoms return or worsen.

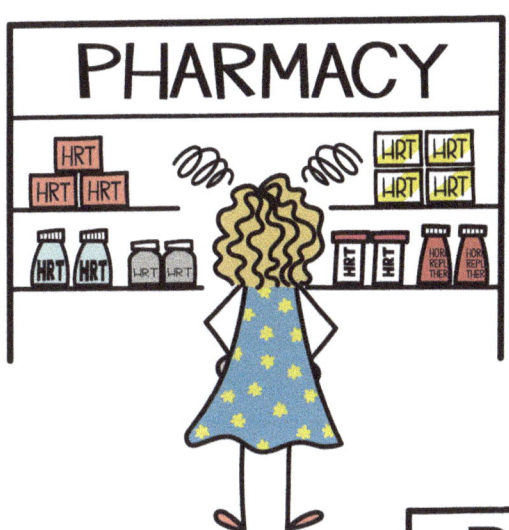
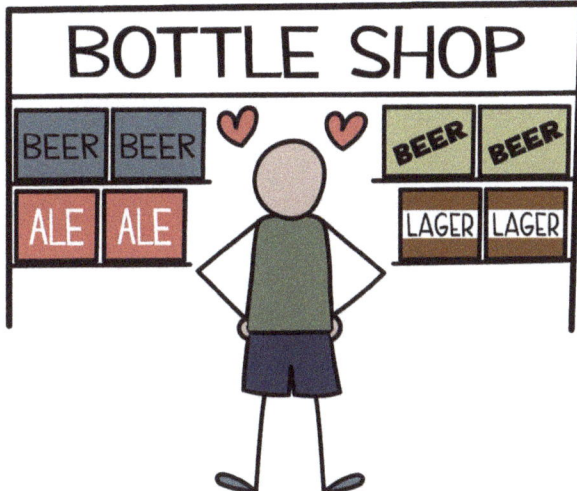

Detailed Definitions

Perimenopause, the transitional phase leading up to menopause. It can last from a few months to up to a decade. On average women experience perimenopause for 4-8 years, which culminates at menopause.

Perimenopause is characterised by hormonal fluctuations that can cause irregular menstrual cycles, hot flashes, sleep disturbances, mood changes, decreased bone density, loss of libido, and many other symptoms, some outlined in this book.

Some women experience few symptoms, and/or just for a short period of time, whereas other women may experience a whole array of symptoms that persist for many years.

Menopause is a specific point in time, diagnosed after a woman has gone 12 consecutive months without menstrual bleeding.

It officially marks the end of fertility and the end of all menstrual cycles.

The average age when menopause occurs, is 51 years old.

Menopause is declared, after the fact of 12 months in amenorrhea*, (if there were no other biological or physiological interventions). However, if the woman has a Uterine Device, or is taking HRT (that prevents periods), or has had a full or partial hysterectomy then a declaration of 'menopause' is not possible by this '12-month menstrual absentee method' alone. A test (or several) for the level of Follicle Stimulating Hormone (FSH) is conducted, usually along with other hormones such as Luteinizing Hormone (LH), and if the woman has FSH levels consistently elevated to 30 mIU/mL or higher, it can confirm menopause.

***Amenorrhea** is the absence of menstrual bleeding.

IMPORTANT: Menopause medical definition vs common language.

Commonly we talk about 'menopause' as the phase over 'x' number of years during which women (may) experience hallmark symptoms. But, by medical definition, women are in perimenopause when they are experiencing such symptoms, right up to the point and inclusive of, the final 12 months without a period.

Menopause therefore is actually just the final point of perimenopause (see Fig. 1 The Menopause Timeline) and simply a marker between peri-menopause and post-menopause.

It isn't the era of which we colloquially call 'menopause', or 'being menopausal'.

Post menopause is the phase in a woman's life following menopause (declaration/moment in time). Some symptoms experienced during perimenopause may persist for several more years, but the ongoing absence of a menstrual cycle (and at least one FSH test) confirms being in the post-menopausal stage of life.

Key Hormones

Estrogen, a key female hormone produced mainly by the ovaries, regulates menstrual cycles and reproductive functions. During perimenopause and menopause, estrogen levels fluctuate and decline, leading to symptoms like hot flashes, mood swings, and changes in bone density, marking the transition from reproductive years to menopause, and post menopause.

Progesterone works alongside estrogen to regulate menstrual cycles (and support pregnancy). In the context of perimenopause and menopause, progesterone levels drop as ovulation becomes irregular and eventually ceases, contributing to menstrual irregularities and perimenopause symptoms.

Follicle-Stimulating Hormone (FSH) is a hormone released by the pituitary gland, responsible for stimulating the growth of eggs in the ovaries and regulating the menstrual cycle. During perimenopause, the ovaries gradually cease functioning and produce less estrogen, prompting the pituitary gland to release more FSH in an attempt to stimulate estrogen production. The FSH test for women is a crucial diagnostic tool used to assess menopausal status.

Hormone Replacement Therapy (HRT) is an optional treatment that may alleviate menopausal symptoms and prevent osteoporosis by supplementing estrogen, progesterone, or both, tailored for women undergoing menopause or perimenopause to balance hormonal levels and enhance quality of life.

Role of Estrogen in HRT: Estrogen is the key hormone in HRT, often the sole hormone used to manage menopause-related symptoms and prevent osteoporosis. By replenishing decreased estrogen levels, it addresses symptoms and mitigates long-term risks like bone density loss. The inclusion of estrogen, and in some cases exclusively, is tailored based on individual health profiles, balancing its significant benefits against potential risks to ensure effective perimenopause management.

Estrogen(s) that make up HRT: Estrogens that may be used in hormone therapies encompass synthetic estrogen, bioidentical estrogen from plant sources, conjugated estrogens from pregnant horse urine, and estrogen esters, which are metabolised into natural estrogen in the body.

Role of Progesterone in HRT: A woman might take progesterone as part of HRT to balance the effects of estrogen, especially if she still has her uterus. Estrogen alone can thicken the uterine lining, increasing the risk of endometrial cancer. Progesterone helps counteract this by thinning the lining, reducing the cancer risk. Additionally, progesterone can help alleviate perimenopausal symptoms, like irregular periods and mood swings, making it a crucial component of HRT for overall hormonal balance and symptom management.

Progesterone(s) that make up HRT: In HRT, various forms of progesterone or progestogens are used to complement estrogen therapy for women with a uterus intact, including natural progesterone from plant sources, synthetic progestins like medroxyprogesterone acetate, and micronised progesterone for enhanced absorption.

Hot Flashes/Hot Flushes: A hot flash (or hot flush as some people prefer to call it) is a sudden, intense feeling of heat that typically originates in the upper body or face, spreading downwards and often leading to sweating, redness, and a rapid heartbeat. Common during perimenopause and caused by hormonal changes affecting the body's temperature regulation. Hot flashes can vary in frequency and intensity, sometimes followed by chills or a cooling sensation.

Epilogue

Post these challenging years of infrequent sex, random rants, excessive body heat, unexpected crying, enlarged boobs and belly, and sometimes just a general 'WTF?', there emerges Woman 2.0.

The upgraded version will enjoy intimacy again, have conversations without tears, and resume a genuine interest in life and the people around her.

So don't despair; perimenopause is a transitional time, and you can both make it through and be stronger as a couple than before. With a little understanding from the XY chromosome partner and a bit of patience, the era of She-Rex will become extinct.

Here's a short list of what you can hope for after the maelstrom:

- Calmness
- Desire to travel
- Fun, joy, and laughter
- Genuine lovemaking and some hot, uninhibited sex
- Joint projects (not just knee replacements!)
- Creativity
- Optimism
- More respect for each other and your aging bodies
- Sleep—oh, blessed sleep—and equity in mattress real estate
- Cuddles that last longer than the next hot flash
- Activities and exercise you both enjoy
- Deep gratitude that you supported her through 'the change'.

There is light and life at the end of the tunnel! You two have got this!

Acknowledgements

My loyal and loving partner Matt, had it not been for you, this book would never have been conceived, let alone completed. I wish to thank you with all my heart for your unwavering belief in me, as well as your input into the content and context of this book. Above all, I am deeply thankful for your patience, care, and support as I traversed through the turbulence of perimenopause.

I would like to thank my daughter, Hanna-Jane, who, despite having a grumpy, tired, emotional, and (now) overweight mum, continues to reassure me that I am still beautiful, lovable, loving, and capable. She also makes me laugh often, which probably keeps me sane.

I would like to praise Kylie Dunn for her wonderful gift in creating the very relatable illustrations from my scratched-out stick figures and for crafting this whole thing into a bedside book for couples to enjoy and benefit from, and for me to be proud of.

I am very grateful to my key editor and forever 'beau-tea-ful' friend, Judy. We spent invaluable hours discussing perimenopause, books, podcasts, and our own symptoms. We share the view that women are not given advanced warning nor an informative booklet by their healthcare providers about this significant phase of aging.

Lastly, I wish to thank my two local besties, Carolyn and Mikala, who read my first draft and gave me food for thought on the target audience, which ultimately changed this book from being a 'Man's Guide…' to a 'Couple's Guide…'. Beyond that, they continued to provide love, encouragement, gin, and giggles!

And to anyone else, including family, friends, and employees, who have put up with an irritable, forgetful, fatigued, middle-aged Samantha … thank-you!

About the Author

Samantha Siân Brown is a former Senior Environmental Scientist and proud owner of a successful tea business in Tasmania, Australia. She has a teenage daughter and two indoor, free-to-roam bunnies.

In her mid-40s, Samantha found herself struggling with the demands of running a business, parenting a very sporty teenager, incessant joint pain, broken sleep, rapid weight gain, and an unusually low libido. Perimenopause was the culprit.

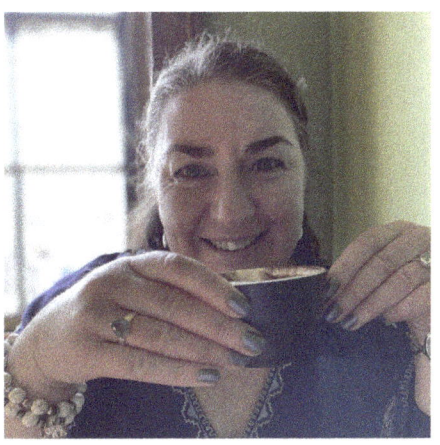

Confused, tired, and frustrated by her ever-changing physical and mental landscape, she wished she had a 'Short Guide' to help explain her roller coaster of moods, weight change, unwieldy periods, interrupted sleep, and many other symptoms to her caring and supportive partner, Matt.

With a desire to help others, a hunger for knowledge, and an ambition to one day write a book, she used her direct experience with perimenopause, a background in science supplemented by contemporary research and a sense of humour to create this unique guidebook.

www.ingramcontent.com/pod-product-compliance
Lightning Source LLC
Chambersburg PA
CBHW040821040426
42333CB00065B/3375